DIALYSIS

and the

RENAL DIET

AVOID THESE 7 MISTAKES,

GET READY TO FEEL BETTER AND HAVE

MORE ENERGY

Sue Emeny

Paperback ISBN: 978-0-9886815-9-0
PDF ISBN: 979-8-9988611-3-0
EPUB ISBN: 978-0-9886815-8-3

https://KidneyDietCentral.com

S.A.G.E. Publishing
P.O.B. 214
Canastota, NY 13032

To my husband Bill, my best friend and the love of my life.
He is why I am still alive today

Contents

Introduction 1

Rediscover Your Favorite Foods 3

Avoiding Nutritional Pitfalls 7

The Vital Importance of a Renal Diet 11

Enhancing Your Dialysis Journey 17

Overcoming the Fluid Removal Challenge 23

The Overlooked Danger of Potassium Depletion 29

Navigating the Dosage Dilemma: Avoiding the Pitfalls of
Overmedication 33

BONUS: How to Make Your Doctor Listen 37

BONUS: The 5 Dialysis Secrets That Can Save Your Life 43

Conclusion 49

About the Author 51

Unlock the Delicious Secrets to a Healthier You 53

Appendix A: Glossary 55

Appendix B FAQs 59

Appendix C Resources 65

Appendix D: Endnotes 67

Introduction

I f you're reading this, then you've just purchased my book "*Dialysis and the Renal Diet*," and I am so happy to have you aboard! As someone who was on dialysis for 8 years, I know how difficult the process can be and how overwhelming it can seem. That's why I wrote this book – to provide practical advice so you can have a better quality of life while on dialysis.

This book is your go-to guide for mastering dialysis and the renal diet. Not only will you learn the mistakes to avoid, but I'll also provide you with examples, advice, and tools to help you on your journey. I've tried it all and figured out how to make dialysis work for me – now I'm here to help you do the same.

I bet when you were first diagnosed with kidney failure, you were or are like a deer in headlights. You were wondering which way to turn and what to do, and you probably didn't even know what questions to ask. You might have been (or are) just a bit scared. In this book, I will try to answer those questions, including those you have yet to learn about. I will also give you the best information I can about dialysis, the renal diet, and their relationship.

At the end of this book, you'll be equipped with the knowledge and confidence to take the steps you need to have a better quality of life. You'll better understand the process and be able to make informed decisions about your health and lifestyle. I'm excited to be a part of your journey, and I'm here to guide you every step of the way.

You've got the book, so what are you waiting for? It's time to get started! Read it with an open mind, and I promise you'll be amazed at the positive changes you start to notice. Dialysis doesn't have to be a burden – it can be a tool to help you live a happy, healthy life, just like it did for me.

Conquer Dialysis and Diet with Sue

When I was diagnosed with renal failure in 2012, I was determined to make the best of my situation. Despite the fact that I had to start dialysis and follow a strict renal diet, I refused to let it stop me from living a full life. I took it upon myself to use my research and engineering skills to determine the best form of dialysis for me and how to make following a renal diet easier.

I have written *Dialysis and the Renal Diet* to help others with renal failure live a normal life while on dialysis. I have used my engineering skills and real-life experience to create a comprehensive guide that will help you take control of your dialysis and diet. I hope to inspire you to take control of your diet and live a good quality of life while on dialysis, just as I did.

If you have renal failure and are looking for help with diet and information on dialysis, then continue reading. You'll be amazed at what a normal life you can lead!

I believe in you, and I know you can do this. Good luck!

Rediscover Your Favorite Foods

Don't Let Dietary Restrictions Stop You from Enjoying Food!

When you are first diagnosed with kidney failure and have to start dialysis, you have to learn about kidney diets and their restrictions; it is a difficult time for many people. One of the biggest mistakes dialysis newbies make is the belief that they cannot eat their favorite foods ever again; this can be very depressing. The truth is that you will be able to eat these foods again as soon as you learn how to keep track of the nutrients you are eating. It is important to remember that a varied diet, including fruits and vegetables, is key to maintaining good health.

Dialysis newbies often make this mistake because the renal diet is introduced through confusing restriction-based lists, not practical guidance on what actually works day to day. Patients are told what to limit—but not how to turn those limits into real meals they can live with.

Most newbies, including myself, when I was a newbie, suffer from the false belief that if a food is "high" in potassium, phosphorus, or sodium, then that food is forbidden. For example, I love pasta; it is a comfort food for me. But spaghetti sauce is "high" in potassium, so I believed I had to give it up. I did give up pasta for a short while until I discovered the secret of tracking nutrients.

Giving up certain foods is a mistake; sadly, most people don't even know they are making this mistake. Learning how to follow a renal diet properly will allow you to eat the food you

3

like, even if it's on the list of restricted or forbidden foods. Doing this can help you maintain your health without feeling deprived.

While you are learning how to follow a renal diet, ask your dietitian for some sample recipes or meal plans. Better yet, "_The Dialysis Patients' Magic Recipe Cookbook (Appendix C)_" contains meal plans and recipes. It will also teach you how to follow a renal diet.

Consequences of Giving Up Particular Foods Unnecessarily.

You will likely feel deprived if you give up the food you like and enjoy eating. This happens to weight loss dieters as well. It is doubtful that you can follow a diet and stay on it for any length of time if you feel deprived and consequently depressed. If you are anything like me, you will probably throw up your hands and say, "The heck with it!" This is not a good thing.

However, just because you don't give up a particular food doesn't mean you can eat all you want of that food. **Eating too much of a restricted food will likely make you feel nauseous and make dialysis side effects harsher.**

Let me tell you a quick story:

> _I was happily living, enjoying all my favorite comfort food and feeling fantastic. Then, my kidneys failed. I had to go on dialysis and give up all my favorite foods. At the time, I had no idea how much this would impact my life. I was clueless and felt lost with all the confusing diet instructions._
>
> _Just when I thought things couldn't get worse, I started to pore over my diet lists, looking for foods I could eat. Every time I found something low in one nutrient, it was high in another. I hit rock bottom when I realized I could no longer eat spaghetti, chili, or tacos, foods I loved. I broke down in tears, feeling like I couldn't eat anything at all._

But then, seeing me cry, my husband stepped in and helped me figure out the diet. He realized that we needed real numbers describing my diet. My dietitian had not yet given me this information.

Suddenly, I had a new spark of hope. I knew what I had to do. I had to get those numbers and practice portion control!

My #1 Piece of Advice

Here's the best piece of advice I have for dialysis newbies: use **portion control**! Don't completely give up the food you love. It's tempting to cut out all the foods you love when you first begin dialysis, but it's important to remember that portion control is the key to eating the food you love.

It's also important to remember that dialysis doesn't have to mean giving up all of your favorite treats. Even with dialysis, you can still enjoy a small slice of cake or a scoop of ice cream occasionally. **Moderation is essential**, and so is keeping track of the nutrients you are eating. Speaking with your dietitian before making any drastic changes to your diet is vital.

Remember:

❦ Giving up your favorite food is detrimental to your soul and spirit, and not necessary

❦ Portion control is the key to eating your favorite foods

Now that you understand the mistake of unnecessarily giving up certain foods, it is just as vital to understand the importance of having a daily nutritional budget to maintain a kidney-friendly diet

Avoiding Nutritional Pitfalls

Lack of Clear Nutritional Limits is a Big Mistake

When it comes to dialysis, there's a lot to learn. You need to know the maximum amount of potassium, phosphorus, sodium, and fluid you can consume each day. Many dialysis patients make the mistake of not having clear nutritional limits. It's a mistake that can lead to difficulties with dialysis, such as cramping and nausea.

Eating without nutritional limits leads to severe health complications like high blood pressure, fluid retention, and nausea, among others. To stay healthy, it's essential to understand how to eat, not what you can and can't eat.

There are a couple of reasons why people on dialysis make this mistake. First, they may not be aware of the importance of their diet. Secondly, they may be overwhelmed by the confusing information about diet and nutrition and need help understanding it.

When you first start dialysis, you may be so focused on getting through the process that you don't know where to turn for answers about following a renal diet.

So, what should you do? It's essential to work with your doctor and dietitian to come up with a plan that works for you. This plan should include specific daily potassium, phosphorus, sodium, and fluid limits.

For instance, my daily limits were:

- Potassium   2,000 milligrams (mg.)
- Phosphorus 1,000 mg.
- Sodium 2,000 mg.
- Fluid   1 liter

Making sure you have clear daily nutritional limits is critical for you to live a good life while on dialysis. It's necessary to know how to eat. Doing so can help you stay healthy and enjoy the benefits of dialysis without the harsh side effects. You must also speak with your doctor or dietitian if you have any questions.

Consequences of Not Having Daily Nutritional Limits

You may not realize you need daily nutritional limits when you start dialysis, but the consequences could be much worse than you think. With a daily dietary budget, you can avoid too much phosphorus, potassium, sodium, or water, which can cause dangerous health problems. For example, eating too much potassium can cause it to build up in your bloodstream and cause serious heart problems, even a heart attack. It can even be life-threatening. Too much phosphorus will make you itch and calcify your organs over time, a deadly consequence! So, it's critical to make sure you have daily nutrition limits and stay within them to stay healthy and safe.

What Should You Do?

You need to have daily nutrition limits, so your best bet is to ask your dietitian for them. Once you have your daily nutrition limits and you start tracking what you eat, you can adjust what and how much you eat to stay within those limits. **This will help you feel your best after a dialysis session and is likely to positively affect your dialysis prescription.**

Tools To Get the Job Done Faster, Better, Easier

Kidney Diet Central offers tools to help you gather nutritional information and track your diet.

- *The Dialysis Patient's Magic Recipe Cookbook in Appendix C* will walk you through the "how to" of following a renal diet.

- *The Kidney Food Finder in Appendix C* is a push-button software that is the quick, easy, and simple solution for finding the nutritional values of your food.

My #1 Piece of Advice

My best advice when it comes to dialysis is to always know your daily nutritional limits and stay within them. You need to be aware of the amount of sodium, potassium, phosphorus, and fluid you consume daily. Monitoring these levels will help you avoid potential health complications, such as heart problems and calcified organs.

I encourage you to take action on this advice by speaking to your doctor or dietitian about your daily nutritional limits. They can help you determine the right balance of nutrients for your unique needs and help you stick to your dietary goals. It is essential to check with your doctor or nurse before making any changes to your diet or lifestyle.

Daily nutritional limits allow you to keep your dialysis treatments successful. They help you to feel better during and after each treatment. So, take the time to talk to your healthcare provider and take control of your diet today.

Remember

- Establish a plan with a dietitian to create personalized nutrition goals

- Monitor potassium, phosphorus, and sodium levels

- Track your daily totals of phosphorus, potassium, sodium, and fluids

- Show these totals to your doctor.

Daily nutritional limits are essential in managing your health; not following a renal diet is detrimental to your health and well-being. Let's explore why following a renal diet is so critical.

The Vital Importance of a Renal Diet

The Mistake of Not Following a Renal Diet

S tarting dialysis can be a difficult adjustment for many people, and one mistake that dialysis newbies often make is not following a renal diet. A renal diet is specifically tailored to meet the dietary needs of those with kidney disease. Not following a renal diet can have serious consequences, and understanding why it is essential is the first step toward better health.

Quality of life is a big issue when you are dealing with kidney failure and dialysis. A direct relationship exists between diet, dialysis treatment, quality of life, and overall well-being.

You or anybody facing or experiencing dialysis must understand the connection between their diet, lab results, dialysis prescription, and how they feel after treatment. By doing so, you are more likely to experience a better quality of life and be able to eat a larger variety of foods or more significant portions.

When the kidneys stop working properly or cease to function altogether, dialysis plays a vital role. It helps remove toxins from the body and keeps fluids, potassium, phosphorus, and sodium (salt) at their proper levels.

Dialysis is not easy on your body. If you bust your daily limits, you will have high blood levels of potassium, phosphorus, sodium, and fluid, making you feel nauseous. The increased blood levels will require more dialysis by increasing the dialysis time, speed, or both.

More dialysis over the same amount of time is harsher on your body and can cause nasty side effects and long-term consequences, including organ calcification and a heart attack.

While on dialysis, you will have a prescription that defines how much fluid and other nutrients will be removed from your blood. The more you eat over your dietary limits, the more that has to be removed. This makes the treatment harsher, making you feel worse when it is done. The more fluid that has to be removed means that you will have to dialyze longer or remove liquid faster. The faster you remove fluid, the worse you are going to feel.

You might not follow a renal diet if you don't fully understand why it is critical to your well-being. You may also need help finding answers, so read on; the answers are in this book.

There are also those people who do not realize the importance of a renal diet. When they start to experience the health issues that can arise from not following one, they wonder why they feel so bad. They also often wonder why their doctor doesn't help them. I talk about that in a later chapter.

Consequences of Not Following a Renal Diet.

As I said before, the consequences can be dire if you do not follow a renal diet. Not following a renal diet can lead to several health issues, which include an increased risk of developing softened bones, calcified organs, heart problems, and even a heart attack. These serious medical issues can be avoided by following a renal diet. And here's the thing: These consequences are MUCH worse than you think because they're not just temporary issues. They can stay with you for life, affecting your quality of life and leading to an earlier death. So, if you're on dialysis, following your renal diet is necessary to avoid these severe risks.

What Should You Do?

A renal dietitian can and should provide you with personalized nutrition advice to help you meet your specific needs. They can also teach you to read food labels and choose the right foods and meal plans. This is the absolute best option because they have specialized knowledge in renal nutrition and can provide tailored advice to meet your needs. Remember, you must ask your dietitian for your daily dietary budget.

To put this into immediate action, you can:

1. Get your daily nutritional limits from your dietitian.

2. Look up the nutritional value of your food.

3. Weigh your food to determine how much potassium, phosphorus, sodium, and water are in your food serving.

4. Read food labels carefully and be aware of the sodium, phosphorus, and potassium content.

5. Use small portions of foods with a lot of potassium, phosphorus, sodium, or water.

6. Keep a running total of each nutrient for the day.

7. Keep a food diary to show your doctor; it will help him adjust your dialysis prescription to your unique needs.

8. Do NOT exceed your daily limits!

9. Ask questions if you're unsure about anything.

What Else to Be Aware Of?

1. Many people think they cook without salt because they don't use a salt shaker. The condiments you may use in your cooking often contain a lot of salt. For example, Worcestershire sauce, soy sauce, ketchup, and blended spices like chili powder or poultry seasoning.

2. When buying meat, especially poultry or pork, look for signs that the meat has been "flavor enhanced" or "tenderized." This usually means the meat has been injected with a 12-15% saline solution. In other words, extra salt and fluid!

3. Avoid adding extra salt to food.

4. Avoid processed (deli meat) and packaged foods, as they are high in sodium and phosphates.

5. Look for "phos" in any ingredient because it is a form of phosphorus.

6. Don't be afraid to ask your dietitian or doctor any questions you may have.

7. Remember that your diet plays a crucial role in your overall dialysis treatment.

8. Watch out for salt substitutes that contain potassium.

9. Lastly, stay motivated and don't lose sight of the long-term benefits of a renal diet.

My #1 Piece of Advice

My most significant piece of advice for dialysis newbies is to be sure to follow a renal diet. This is necessary! Eating right is a crucial part of dialysis care, and it can make a big difference in how you feel, especially after a dialysis session. A renal diet can help you keep your potassium, phosphorus, and sodium levels in check.

I encourage you to take action now and learn all you can about creating and following a renal diet. Eating right is essential to dialysis care, and you'll be glad you took the time to learn how to eat on a renal diet. You can find detailed information in the book, _The Dialysis Patient's Magic Recipe Cookbook in Appendix C._

Remember

🙟 Speak with a renal dietitian for a personalized plan.

🙟 Read labels and be aware of the sodium content of foods.

🙟 Beware of any ingredient with the "phos" in the name.

🙟 Avoid added salt, processed, and packaged foods.

Now that we understand the consequences of not following a renal diet let's examine how not understanding the link between diet and dialysis can further complicate a patient's journey with failed kidneys.

Dialysis and the Renal Diet

Enhancing Your Dialysis Journey

The Essential Role of Diet: Why underestimating the power of your diet is a mistake

You may be making a significant mistake without even realizing it when it comes to dialysis. Failing to understand the impact of diet on dialysis is a massive mistake with severe consequences, such as decreased quality of life and other health complications. Here's why it's such a big mistake.

If you want to feel the best that you can while on dialysis, then following a renal diet is necessary. You need to adjust your diet according to your dialysis prescription. It is essential and rewarding.

The link between diet and dialysis is an important one. Dialysis is an artificial process that helps to remove excess nutrients, toxins, and fluid from your body. The foods you eat can affect the amount of these elements you need to remove.

Dialysis is a fixed process; you do it the same way every time. How can you expect good results if you eat however much you want of whatever you want? The answer is that you can't—and you can't blame your doctor because he can only prescribe a fixed process based on your lab results, which probably change monthly if you are not watching your diet closely.

Doctors prescribe your dialysis, while dietitians prescribe your diet. The connection between diet and dialysis is rarely explained. Newbies and even veterans are often unaware of the relationship between what they eat and how it affects their dialysis and overall well-being. They suffer from this lack of knowledge.

17

By learning more about the importance of your diet, you can minimize the unwanted side effects of dialysis and feel better after treatment.

Consequences of Not Understanding the Link Between Diet and Dialysis.

If your diet does not match your dialysis prescription, you may experience severe fatigue or muscle cramps during or after treatment. I have heard people groan or scream in pain from severe cramping during an in-center dialysis treatment. More than once, I left the dialysis center exhausted and needed to go home and sleep.

You need to be aware of the possible buildup of excess fluid in your body, which can lead to swelling, trouble breathing, and heart problems. Not to mention that not removing sufficient phosphorus during dialysis treatment can lead to severe itching and calcified organs.

It is essential to understand the relationship between diet and dialysis, and **it is important to follow a diet that matches your dialysis prescription.**

When you're new to dialysis, it's common to miss the connection between your diet and treatment results. Many people begin by restricting fluids and avoiding certain foods to try to improve their condition, but these aren't always the best solutions.

As mentioned previously, continuously depriving yourself of foods you love can make you depressed, and you may not want to bother with it all. Take heart. You really don't have to deprive yourself completely. The best way to bridge the gap between diet and dialysis is to work with your doctor and dietitian to develop a personalized plan that matches your diet to your dialysis treatment. I'll explain more about this in a later chapter.

How Do You Know If You Have a Good Diet?

There are two strong reasons to believe that you follow a good diet that matches your dialysis prescription. The first reason is that your lab results are **all** in their proper range. The second reason is that you **feel good**. If you don't feel good and have good lab results, there is something wrong with your dialysis prescription. When this happened to me, I had a very difficult time convincing my doctor that he needed to do something about the dialysis prescription.

Kidney patients must maintain constant daily nutrition levels so their doctor can better evaluate their lab results. *The doctor has to decide whether the diet or the prescription is causing the unsatisfactory lab results and causing you to feel lousy.*

If you have received your daily nutrition limits from your dietitian for your type of dialysis, then you've already taken the first step toward maintaining your nutrition levels. Next, start tracking the food you eat by weighing or measuring everything you consume and keeping a daily running total. Now, you have the information you need to use portion control to keep within your daily limits.

When you show your food log to your doctor, he can adjust your dialysis prescription to match your diet or suggest changes to your diet.

If you do not pay attention to nutrition and fluids, you will probably end up with a one-size-fits-all prescription and not get the attention you need to eventually feel better.

My experience with dialysis showed me that tracking my nutrition gave me a better chance of convincing my doctor to make changes. I found him to be more willing to work with me toward my ultimate goal of feeling better and increasing my life expectancy.

By tracking your diet, you show your doctor that you care about yourself and are paying attention. Your doctor will then be more apt to recommend you for a transplant when he knows that you are paying attention and doing what you need to do to feel better.

My experience has also shown me that you must **advocate** for yourself and convince your doctors to make a change to help you feel better.

Let me tell you a secret: you can have great lab results and still feel lousy. I had great lab results for 4 ½ years and felt awful for 3 ½ years, even though I was religiously following my renal diet! I finally asked my doctor, "*If my labs are so good, why do I feel so bad?*"

This is a crucial question! Your lab results will guide doctors, but many will not consider how you feel. It stopped my doctor dead in his tracks. He was on his way out the door as I asked the question. He stopped, turned around, and started discussing the problem with me.

He moved me from 3 days a week to every other day. It helped, but I still felt terrible after treatment and felt awful for the rest of the day. He then moved me to 5 times a week. My lab results stayed within range the whole time, and I began to feel alive again!

When you use the nutrition data to follow your diet closely, you will have good lab results to show your doctor at your monthly visit, and he will have more information to help him prescribe the best dialysis prescription for you.

How to Get the Nutrition Data You Need

Food Data Central (Appendix C) is a free, online nutrition database from the U.S. Department of Agriculture. While it contains extensive nutrition data, it is not user-friendly. Finding the right food entry can be tedious and overwhelming, making it a poor day-to-day tool for people trying to manage a kidney diet.

Kidney Diet Central provides practical, affordable software that turns nutrition data into usable information. *Kidney Food Finder*

(Appendix C) allows users to instantly see protein, phosphorus, potassium, and sodium values and adjust portion sizes to fit their real-life diet.

By removing guesswork and frustration, Kidney Food Finder makes it far easier to follow a kidney-friendly diet. What once took long searches through complex databases can now be done in seconds. Although built for people with kidney failure, the software also works well for people with diabetes and anyone who wants better control over what they eat.

My #1 Piece of Advice

Here is my primary advice: respect the relationship between diet and dialysis. It's critical to your long-term health and well-being.

Remember:

- Keeping your doctor informed of your diet will help him to adjust your dialysis prescription to your specific needs.
- Kidney patients must maintain constant daily nutrition levels to evaluate lab results better.
- *Kidney Food Finder (Appendix C)* is inexpensive software that makes tracking nutrition and fluids easy.

Given the importance of controlling fluid levels during dialysis, it is essential to understand the connection between diet and dialysis to ensure the patient's safety. In the next chapter, we will begin exploring mistakes concerning your dialysis treatment.

Dialysis and the Renal Diet

Overcoming the Fluid Removal Challenge

Your Essential Guide to Safe Dialysis Practices

B efore we start talking about the fluid removal part of dialysis, you need to understand the concept of *dry weight*. Your dry weight is your weight when you are not retaining water. Often, it is what you weighed before your kidneys failed.

When you start dialysis, you, your doctor, and/or your medical team will decide your dry weight; this is an important number. The amount of fluid that is removed from your body during dialysis is calculated as the difference between your current weight and your dry weight. This is the amount of fluid you have retained since the last time you dialyzed.

How Much Fluid Should You Remove?

If you know how much fluid you put on, then you know how much fluid you should remove during dialysis; this is a good reason to monitor how much you drink. It is crucial to remove the right amount of fluid during dialysis. Not removing enough fluid can cause swelling and high blood pressure. Removing too much fluid can cause dizziness, low blood pressure, and muscle cramps; you might even faint.

Not drinking all the coffee and water you want is a hard change to get used to; at least, it was for me. If you want to feel the best you can after dialysis, limit your fluid intake; for me, it was about one liter a day. It is hard to do for many people, but you will find that it is worthwhile, especially if you are going to a center or hospital for dialysis.

Let me tell you a story about when I was dialyzing in-center.

> *I got really sick and ended up in the hospital for about four days. I had an IV drip; they fed me the wrong food for a person on dialysis, and, of course, I didn't pee. I gained twenty pounds, which is roughly nine liters; I felt horrible. When I finally got out of the hospital and went to the center to dialyze, I said, "Just take it all off."*

> *They wouldn't do it. They told me that three liters is the most fluid they would remove at one time. I had to drink less than they could remove between sessions, or I wouldn't lose the excess fluid. It was hard drinking so little, but I eventually got rid of the excess without suffering from low blood pressure, dizziness, or cramping.*

Why The Three-Liter Max?

The dialysis machine can only remove water from your blood. Any excess water you may retain, such as the twenty pounds I mentioned, is stored within and between your cells. As the water is removed from your blood, water will *slowly* migrate from your body cells into your blood.

Depending on size, adults contain about four to six liters of blood. So, as you can see, there is no way I could have removed nine liters of fluid.

But what happens if I remove three liters? I'm still going to feel tired and drained. I might even get cramps. If I have six liters of blood in my body, three liters is one-half of my blood. This is why it is important to limit your fluid intake. After this experience, I limited myself to drinking one liter of fluid a day. It was hard!

Why is "removing too much fluid too fast" a mistake?

Removing too much fluid too fast during dialysis is a common mistake made by many people. This happens when you drink too much between dialysis sessions. Since you don't urinate, dialysis is the only way to remove excess fluid from your body. This means you must be careful how much you drink. That is why I limited myself to two liters or less between sessions.

Most people starting on dialysis make the mistake of not linking the amount of fluid they drink in a day to how much fluid dialysis can remove in one session. Remember, the more fluid you remove, the worse you will feel after dialysis.

When I was on in-center dialysis, I limited my fluid intake to one liter a day; it was difficult drinking so little and not drinking all that I wanted, but it made dialysis easier.

Consequences of removing too much fluid too fast.

If you make the mistake of removing too much fluid too fast, besides making you feel lousy, the consequences can be dire. Your blood pressure could drop dangerously low, and the chance of a heart attack or stroke increases. In addition, the sudden change in fluid levels of your blood can cause severe headaches, nausea, cramping, and fatigue.

The removal of water from your blood also causes electrolytes (potassium and sodium) to be removed. This leads to severe cramping and heart problems. It is essential to stay within the safe limits of fluid removal while undergoing dialysis; the consequences of not doing so can be much worse than you think.

What Should You Do?

The best way to avoid this mistake is **not to drink very much!**

Measure your fluid intake so you know how much you are drinking. I allowed myself 1 ½ liters of fluid daily when I was on home dialysis and was dialyzing five times a week; only 1 liter when I was dialyzing in-center. Of course, the amount I allowed myself to drink was tied to my dialysis prescription.

Limiting your daily fluid intake is the easiest way to avoid the mistake of having to remove too much fluid too fast. If you are not dialyzing in-center, you can also lengthen your dialysis session or increase the number of sessions to remove excess fluid safely. Here's how you can manage your fluid intake:

1. Buy a small scale or use a measuring cup to keep track of how much fluid you drink.

2. Keep a diary of your fluid intake throughout the day. Stop drinking when you reach one liter.

3. Weigh yourself before and after dialysis to accurately assess how much fluid you have removed. Strive to reach your dry weight each time.

4. Monitor your body weight daily and make any necessary adjustments to your fluid intake.

5. Remember there is a lot of fluid in soups, boiled food, and many other foods.

These tips will help you measure and take control of your fluid intake. This will help you avoid removing too much fluid too fast and suffering the consequences.

How To Fix the Mistake If You Have Already Made It

You cannot do much if you do dialysis in a center. You can insist that the dialysis techs do not remove too much fluid. You are the boss! Have your doctor talk to them if they refuse to listen to you.

Sue Emeny

The best way to fix this mistake is to limit your fluid intake. If you do, you won't have to remove too much fluid too quickly.

If you qualify, a better option is to do dialysis at home.

As potassium depletion can lead to even more severe consequences than removing too much fluid too fast, it is essential to understand how to manage it properly and prevent it from occurring. In the next chapter, we will explore the critical implications of potassium depletion and how to avoid it.

The Overlooked Danger
of Potassium Depletion

E veryone on dialysis should be aware of the overlooked danger of potassium depletion. Potassium depletion in the blood is caused by the dialysis machine removing too much potassium during dialysis treatment. This could result in dangerously low potassium levels in your bloodstream.

Potassium depletion in the blood is a significant reason for the ugly side effects of dialysis treatments. It is a grave mistake because it can lead to various dangerous health conditions, such as fatigue, muscle weakness, irregular heartbeat, and cardiac arrest.

According to Harvard Health[1]:

> *Normal body levels of potassium are important for muscle function. Potassium relaxes the walls of the blood vessels, lowering blood pressure and protecting against muscle cramping. A number of studies have shown an association between low potassium intake and increased blood pressure and higher risk of stroke.*

The link to the full article, "Potassium Lowers Blood Pressure" is in the *Endnotes*.

Therefore, you must be aware of the dangers of potassium depletion and take steps to prevent it. Unfortunately, many dialysis patients suffer from the consequences of potassium depletion without recognizing it. I know I did, and it was several years of doing home dialysis before I discovered what was making me feel bad when I was nearly done dialyzing.

Many people have high levels of potassium, so doctors focus on that. They prescribe a dialysate that removes a lot of potassium. It is often too much when you add the potassium pulled off by the water removal. The same way a bad case of diarrhea requires drinking a lot and replacing your electrolytes.

To avoid this mistake, you should ask your doctor why you feel so bad when you have good lab results. Make sure to tell them when you feel your worst.

A quick story:

In June 2014, my life improved when I began home hemodialysis. A few months later, when a new doctor joined my clinic, the improvement became even more significant. He looked into why I felt so bad, especially after dialysis, and changed my schedule from three days to every other day. Although this helped, I felt terrible after my sessions and the rest of the day. My lab results were still good, however.

I tracked my nutrition with software and was diligent in using it. My doctor and I started reviewing my potassium levels, which were usually in the low normal range of around 3.1 or 3.2. He instructed me to increase my potassium intake from 2000 milligrams a day to 3000 milligrams; my potassium level jumped to nearly 4. I felt a bit better, but still exhausted at the end of dialysis. Based on my attention to diet and these results, my doctor switched me to a dialysate solution that would remove less potassium.

My high blood pressure then dropped to a range of 140 to 160 without using blood pressure meds; this is known to happen when potassium is low. He cut back on how much I dialyzed, and my potassium levels went up to 4.6. Even though my doctor felt better about this, I didn't.

After more conversations, we determined that the potassium in my blood was being depleted during dialysis, leading to my exhaustion. He reluctantly prescribed a potassium pill (390 milligrams each), which I took 45 minutes before the end of the session. The difference was remarkable; I could even help make supper after I got off dialysis.

This was a pivotal discovery for me. I now needed to keep my potassium level at around five and take a potassium supplement 45 minutes before the end of my dialysis session. I should note that these upper-limit potassium levels make the doctors very nervous; after all, too much potassium can cause a heart attack.

I did not need to change my prescription after that. I felt great and went back to living my life.

How To Fix This Problem

As my story shows, you must closely track how much potassium you consume daily.

You also have to work closely with your doctor so that you have his trust. He needs to know that you are:

- Paying attention to your diet.
- Following directions.
- Keeping your medical team informed of any changes you make. (I always asked my dialysis team about whatever it was that I wanted to try and got their approval, sometimes with a warning.)
- Talking to him or her about any changes in your diet or medication that may affect potassium levels.
- Gaining and maintaining his trust.

As I mentioned before, you can use the USDA's *Food Data Central* to determine how much potassium is in your food. It is free and web-based, but it is also tedious to use and requires you to do some calculations.

You can also use the *Kidney Food Finder (Appendix C)* to do the same thing. It is effortless and does all the calculations for you. It is inexpensive, but it is not free.

Use one of these tools to help you track your potassium. Keep a daily log of your potassium intake. Show it to your doctor at your monthly visit. It will help him determine if you need a change in your prescription or possibly a potassium supplement.

My #1 Piece Of Advice

Realize that dialysis often removes too much potassium from your blood, which can cause unwanted and dangerous side effects.

Keep track of the amount of potassium you consume daily. Work with your doctor to get your diet and dialysis prescription matched. Remember

- Dialysis often depletes your potassium levels.
- To examine the potassium levels in your monthly labs.
- Tracking the potassium you consume is necessary to fix the problem.
- To discuss any changes in diet or medication with your doctor

Having highlighted the risk of potassium depletion in the blood, it is also essential to be aware of the potential consequences of administering too much medication too quickly, which we will explore in the next chapter

Navigating the Dosage Dilemma: Avoiding the Pitfalls of Overmedication

The perils of too large a dose of medicine

Are you getting too much medicine all at once, particularly regarding epoetin? Epoetin is a hormone that tells your body to build up your hemoglobin. Any medication in too large a dose can cause side effects ranging from mildly annoying to severe.

Let me tell you a story to illustrate this. A few years back, my hemoglobin went down way too low, so my doctor prescribed a weekly dose of 20,000 units of Epogen. Boy, did I get the side effects! I developed a nasal drip, a cough, weakness, and tiredness. I looked up the side effects of a dose of Epogen that was too large. I discovered that I exhibited many of the potential side effects.

My husband and I are both engineers, and we recognized this phenomenon as acting like an "impulse function." Don't worry about the fancy word. I'll explain.

For example, a working aquarium is normally placid, with no ripples or waves, and the fish are calm and unconcerned. Now, gently push on one side of the aquarium, just a little bit. What will happen? With a few ripples, the fish will barely notice, if they notice at all. The aquarium will settle down and become stable quickly. This scenario represents a standard or low dose of medicine.

After the aquarium has settled down and there are no more ripples, rock the aquarium back and forth vigorously. You will get waves, the fish will slosh around, and some might even fall out, and it will take much longer for the aquarium and the fish to settle or become stable. This scenario represents a high dose of medicine.

In the engineering world, this is called an impulse function. You do this to your body when taking a large dose of medicine.

The video *Too Much Medicine Too Fast* demonstrates this problem. The link is in *Appendix C*.

At my husband's and my request, the doctor reduced the dosage to 5,000 units three times a week. It took a while for my body to adjust, but my symptoms went away, my hemoglobin level rose to a respectable level, and finally, my Epogen dosage was reduced, and I felt better.

Be cautious when taking medication in monthly doses (e.g., Aranesp). The monthly amount can easily be too large and cause side effects. If you are already taking a monthly dose that doesn't bother you, stay with it. However, if you experience side effects from it, ask your doctor for a medication that can be given in smaller, more frequent doses and adjusted to meet your specific needs.

What Should You Do?

The #1 way to avoid the mistake of "too much medicine too fast" is to discuss with your doctor the dosage he is prescribing. Ask if the dose is a large one; is it a standard dosage? Even a typical quantity can be too large for some people.

Here's how you can put this into action:

1. Pay attention to how you feel with a new dosage.

2. Notice any changes that seem unrelated, like a runny nose, for instance, or a cough.

3. Make sure you understand exactly what medications you're taking, the dosage, how they should be taken, and why.

4. Ask your doctor questions if you don't understand something.

By understanding your medications, asking questions, and tracking when you're taking them, you will be sure to take the correct dosage and avoid any potential issues.

How To Fix The Mistake If You've Already Made It

The first step to fixing this mistake is recognizing that you have an issue with a dose that is too large.

Contact your doctor immediately, and tell him what you think is wrong. Explain your symptoms and ask if a smaller, more frequent dose might solve the problem. Sometimes, a dosage adjustment may be necessary, or a different type of medication may be recommended.

My #1 Piece Of Advice

My best advice on dialysis is to avoid making the mistake of taking too much medicine too fast. Always pay attention to any changes in how you feel when you start a new medication or an adjustment to a dosage you are already on.

Remember:

- Take medication as prescribed by your doctor.
- Ask your doctor any questions you have about the dosage and timing.
- It is important to be aware of any side effects that may occur.
- Alert your doctor if any side effects arise.

🫘 Keep track of your medication and its effects.

Now that we've explored the mistake of 'too much medicine too fast,' let's delve into the mistake of not having your doctor listen to your concerns; a critical step to ensuring you receive the best care possible.

BONUS:
How to Make Your Doctor Listen

The Key to Better Dialysis Care

When you are brand new to dialysis, it can be a confusing and overwhelming experience. One of the most significant mistakes made is allowing your doctor to get away with not listening to you.

Let me share a little story that taught me the importance of speaking up and asking questions. My parents had a doctor they thought was fantastic when they were younger. But as they aged, they struggled to voice their concerns. Coming from a generation that viewed doctors as all-knowing authorities, they accepted whatever he said.

Things took a turn when I noticed my mom was heavily prescribed opioids for pain, yet the doctor never bothered to investigate why she was in pain. Concerned, I decided to accompany them to a double appointment. First, we had to wait two hours to see him—definitely a red flag.

As the appointment progressed, the doctor seemed distracted and disinterested. I initially stayed quiet, but I couldn't hold back any longer. I started asking him pointed questions: "Why this?" "Why that?" What happened next was surprising. The doctor straightened up, focused, and began to truly engage with us.

This experience taught me a valuable lesson: never underestimate the power of asking questions. Being proactive and standing up for yourself or your loved ones can lead to better care and understanding. It shows that a bit of advocacy can make a big difference!

Why is letting your doctor get away with not listening to you a mistake? Because it's your health and your life, you should always actively participate in all decisions about your care. It's your right to have a say in the type of dialysis you receive and the medications you take.

If your doctor will not answer your questions or pay attention to you when you tell him about any issues you may be experiencing, you're not getting the best care possible.

Why won't your doctor listen to you?

1. Some doctors are arrogant and don't believe that a mere patient can understand anything.

2. Do you talk to your doctor and let him know that you are paying attention? Often, they don't listen to you because they think you are not paying attention or not following directions.

3. Your doctor doesn't trust you.

4. Do you lie to your doctor? Do you tell them you are following directions when you are not? Do you make changes to your prescription without informing your medical team? Believe me, they will know!

5. Take a look at this video, "*You Can Have A Good Doctor!*" in *Appendix C*.

6. Be honest and upfront about everything you do. Your labs will tell the truth anyway, exposing any falsehood.

Unfortunately, some dialysis patients make this mistake because they're intimidated by their doctor. They don't want to ask questions or challenge their doctor's decisions, so they stay silent.

Sue Emeny

Some patients don't feel comfortable asking for clarification of the medical jargon they don't understand. And finally, they may think that their doctor knows best and that they don't need to ask questions. Check out the video "*Does Your Med Team Trust You?*" in *Appendix C*

Many people make this mistake when they first start dialysis and are feeling overwhelmed and scared. They might not even realize they're making a mistake, but it can seriously affect their health and well-being.

So what should you do instead? First, you should realize that it is OK to ask questions of your medical team. Make sure you are aware of your options. Trust your instincts and speak up if your doctor isn't listening.

Make sure your doctor knows what you are eating. Show your doctor how you know how much potassium, phosphorus, sodium, and fluid you are taking in each day. **Your diet has a dramatic effect on your dialysis prescription.**

Don't let your doctor tune you out. As a dialysis patient, you should ask your doctor a lot of questions about your care and what you can do to help yourself feel better. You need to make informed decisions about your care, so you need to learn all you can about dialysis and kidney failure. Make sure you understand your options and feel empowered to speak up for yourself.

Consequences of letting your doctor get away with not listening to you.

If you let your doctor get away with not listening to you, the consequences can be significant. Not only could it lead to a misdiagnosis or a lack of proper treatment, but it could also mean you're missing out on essential information that could make a real difference in your health and quality of life.

For example:

I was given too large a dose of Epogen, which caused the seemingly unrelated side effect of a nasal drip and dry cough. I needed the large quantity, just not all at the same time. After discussing the issue with my doctor, the dosage was spread out to three times a week. The nasal drip and dry cough went away.

If my doctor had not listened, I would have suffered from the nasal drip and cough for as long as I required that dosage. That's why it's so important to make sure your doctor is taking the time to listen to you. If he doesn't, you'll have to endure the consequences.

What Should You Do?

As a dialysis patient, the #1 way to avoid "letting your doctor get away with not listening to you" is by taking an assertive and confident approach to your healthcare. It's important to remember that you know your body better than anyone else, and it's your right to make sure your doctor listens to your concerns and responds appropriately.

Here's how you can take an assertive and confident approach to your healthcare:

- Ask questions and speak up. Don't be afraid to ask your doctor questions and to speak up if you don't understand something. Doctors are smart; they should be able to explain it to you in a way you can understand.

- Do your own research. Learn as much as you can about dialysis, and take the time to understand any questions or concerns you have.

- Be honest. Let your doctor know if you're having trouble following their advice or if something isn't working for you.

- Get a second opinion. If you don't feel like your doctor is listening to you, getting a second opinion is okay.

- You may even need to find a new doctor.

- If you don't understand something, ask questions until it is explained in a way that you do understand.

- If you feel your doctor is giving you too much or too little information, let them know.

- Don't lie to your medical team.

- Don't skip treatments

- Taking an assertive and confident approach to your healthcare is the best way to ensure your doctor listens to you and takes your concerns seriously. Don't be afraid to speak up and make sure that your questions are answered.

My #1 Piece Of Advice

Here's my best advice: don't let your doctor get away with not listening to you. Remembering that you are your best advocate regarding your health is important. You know your body better than anyone else, and it's essential to make sure your doctor considers your needs regarding treatment. Don't be afraid to speak up and ask questions; make sure your doctor listens to your concerns. It's your health, so take charge and ensure you get the best care possible. Don't be afraid to be your own advocate!

Remember

- Speak up and ask questions

- Challenge, politely, your doctor's opinion if it does not feel right

- Ensure that your doctor knows how much potassium, phosphorus, sodium, and fluid you consume daily; show him.

- Keep your doctor informed of any changes you make to your diet.

- Make sure you understand the diagnosis and plan of care

- If you don't feel comfortable, look for a new doctor

BONUS:
The 5 Dialysis Secrets
That Can Save Your Life

I t's easy to make mistakes when you're new to dialysis, but one of the biggest blunders dialysis newbies can make is missing out on the five secrets to mastering dialysis. These five secrets are essential for a successful dialysis experience and avoiding common pitfalls; many dialysis newbies don't know about them or take them into account.

Dialysis newbies need to understand how to properly take care of their dialysis machine, how to get the most out of their dialysis treatments, and how to stay healthy and strong while going through dialysis. The five dialysis secrets provide the information newbies need to do all this and more.

This mistake is usually made when you are first starting dialysis. This is when you are most overwhelmed and unsure of what to do next.

Secret #1 - Residual Function is Valuable

I really, really wish that my doctor had told me how to preserve my residual renal function. I was just told that people on hemodialysis lose it faster. I asked him why. He gave me a vague "just because" kind of answer. He was lucky I didn't have my wits about me then, or I would never have let him get away with it. Unfortunately, I didn't learn about residual function until too late.

What Is Residual Function?

This is pretty easy to answer. It generally refers to the remaining urine output when you begin dialysis. But I firmly believe that, along with urine output, are the other kidney functions that may still function to some degree. While the kidneys are not doing enough, they are still doing something.

Preserving your residual function or urine output is essential because it reduces the amount of fluid and toxins that have to be removed by dialysis. The less dialysis required, the better! And every little bit helps, or as my doctor said, "Every drop is golden". Removing too much fluid or removing it too fast contributes to the loss of residual function. Performing dialysis at home is the best way to preserve your residual function.

Prolong your life! Slow pump rates, frequent dialysis, and avoiding removing too much fluid can prevent the loss of residual function.

Secret #2 – Organ Stunning and Dehydration

Organ stunning is a serious condition that can occur during hemodialysis. It happens when too much fluid and waste are removed from the blood too quickly. This can cause your heart to work harder than it should, which can lead to long-term damage and even death.

High dialysis machine pump rates and fast fluid removal can shorten your lifespan to 5-7 years, by causing organ damage and dehydration. Your blood thickens, making your heart work harder, and your organs starve for oxygen. Home Dialysis Central has an excellent article explaining organ stunning, _Organ Stunning On Hemodialysis: What Is It And What Can You Do?_ The link is in _Appendix C_

Secret #3 – Nocturnal HHD

Are you tired of being tethered to a dialysis center for hours every week? Consider nocturnal home hemodialysis.

Nocturnal home hemodialysis (HHD) allows you to receive dialysis treatments at home while you sleep. This can offer several benefits, including greater flexibility with scheduling, more frequent treatments, reduced dependence on medications, and no dietary restrictions.

Longer and slower fluid and toxin removal will remove the larger molecules like phosphorus. Short dialysis sessions are not able to remove phosphorus as easily.

Studies[2] have shown that people who switch to nocturnal home hemodialysis experience better outcomes, including improved survival rates and reduced hospitalization.

The process is more straightforward than you might think. You and an optional partner receive training from your clinic's home dialysis nurse.

Say goodbye to the limitations of traditional hemodialysis and improve your quality of life with nocturnal home hemodialysis. Talk to your healthcare provider to see if it's right for you.

Secret #4 – Why More Frequent Dialysis is Better

The idea of undergoing multiple dialysis sessions a week may seem overwhelming. Still, **studies**[2] have shown that longer, slower, and more frequent dialysis is easier on the body and can lead to better outcomes for people with kidney failure.

The more often you do dialysis, the better it is for your health. In fact, studies[2] have shown that patients who receive more frequent hemodialysis treatments experience improved blood pressure, better control of anemia, and fewer hospitalizations.

Peritoneal dialysis is a type of dialysis that involves using the patient's own body as a filter. This method allows for greater flexibility in treatment frequency, making it easier to fit into a patient's schedule.

But why does more frequent, longer, and slower dialysis lead to better outcomes? It is simple: the more often waste and excess fluid are removed from your body, the less damage is done to your organs. This means that patients who undergo more frequent dialysis are less likely to experience health complications such as infections, heart disease, and even death.

So, if you're on dialysis, don't settle for the bare minimum. Talk to your healthcare provider about the benefits of more frequent treatments. You deserve the best care possible, and more frequent or prolonged dialysis treatments could be the key to a longer, healthier life.

Secret #5 – Do Not Allow the Use of Contrast Dye

Contrast dye, also known as radiographic contrast media, is a type of substance injected into the body to help produce more precise images during medical imaging studies such as CT scans or MRIs. It is commonly used to help diagnose various medical conditions, including heart disease, cancer, and kidney issues.

Learn from my experience!

I woke up in excruciating pain while doing my overnight automatic peritoneal dialysis. It was October 2013, and I was at home. The pain was so intense that I could barely move. It became clear that I needed to go to the emergency room. My son and husband had to help me to the car, as I was doubled over and could barely walk.

At the hospital, I was given a contrast dye and underwent a CT scan to determine the cause of my unbearable pain. The diagnosis was an infection, and I was immediately given high-powered intravenous antibiotics to combat it. After four long days in the hospital, the infection was finally gone, but my kidney function had been significantly reduced.

A couple of years later, I went to the Cleveland Clinic to be evaluated for a kidney transplant. The medical team insisted on a CT scan with contrast, which I agreed to. Little did I know that this decision would have a devastating impact on my already compromised kidney function. The contrast dye used in the scan ended up eliminating what little residual kidney function I had left. Without any urine production, I now required more frequent and intense dialysis, which made my life even more challenging than before.

The use of contrast dye for my CT scans had caused irreversible damage to my kidneys, resulting in the loss of my remaining kidney function. This taught me a valuable lesson that I want to share with all renal diet beginners: if you have kidney disease, never let anyone use contrast dye for a CT scan or an MRI. This simple decision can have a profound impact on your health and quality of life.

Conclusion

Your life isn't over. Reclaim your well-being.

Congratulations on reading "Dialysis & The Renal Diet" and gaining a much better understanding of how dialysis and nutrition go hand-in-hand! You've made an essential step in improving your quality of life, feeling better, and avoiding feeling horrible most of the time.

You now have the knowledge and understanding of what it takes to successfully incorporate a renal diet into your dialysis care. You know the mistakes to avoid and the practical advice and examples you need to master this important topic. It's time to take action and implement what you just learned.

One of the best ways to get started is with the included "**Cooking For Dialysis: 7-Day Meal Plan With Recipes**." This helpful cookbook has seven days of meal plans that are dialysis-friendly and tailored to a dialysis patient's dietary needs. Each menu is designed to provide enough calories for energy but also contains the right amount of phosphorus, potassium, and sodium for my prescribed case.

The renal diet is the cornerstone of a successful dialysis treatment plan. With the knowledge you've gained and the tools available to you, you can now take the necessary steps to live a healthier life.

The Dialysis Patient's Creed

I will do my best to take care of my body and dialyze in a way that makes me feel good. I will strive to follow a renal diet that supports my dialysis and makes me feel strong and energized. I will be patient with myself and take the time to learn what works best for my body. I will be kind to myself, understanding that dialysis has its challenges, and I will take each day as it comes. I will dialyze with confidence, a positive attitude, and a commitment to my health and well-being.

About the Author

S usan Emeny wrote "**Dialysis and the Renal Diet**" to empower dialysis beginners to seize control of their diets and lives. After personally battling the challenges of kidney failure, Susan is passionate about sharing her hard-won wisdom—so you don't have to make the same mistakes she did. This book isn't just a guide; it's a roadmap to a good life while living with dialysis.

With a deeply personal connection to the subject, Susan had been on dialysis since 2012, accumulating **8 years of insights** and experiences. She's navigated every type of dialysis available at the time, turning her life's challenges into actionable solutions. Coupled with her background as a **software developer and researcher**, Susan combines technical expertise with personal experience to address the intricate relationship between dialysis and diet. She knows the struggles firsthand and has successfully developed strategies to achieve balance and enjoyment in life while requiring dialysis.

Now is the time to take charge! Dive into Susan's book and unlock the vital knowledge that will help you enjoy a fulfilling life while on dialysis. Grab your copy today and start your journey toward a better life, ensuring that your dialysis experience doesn't define you. Don't Just Survive—Thrive!

Say goodbye to the aftermath of dialysis! Discover how a renal diet can improve your life and help you feel your best.

Unlock the Delicious Secrets to a Healthier You

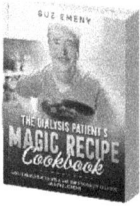

Are you tired of *feeling exhausted and sick* after your dialysis treatments?

Do you wish you could enjoy **mouthwatering meals** without the worry of harming your health? If so, it's time to discover *The Dialysis Patient's Magic Recipe Cookbook!*

Here's What You'll Discover Inside

- **The Renal Diet Simplified**: Easy-to-understand instructions take the mystery out of eating. Safely eat your favorite foods.

- **Tasty Recipes**: Relish in meals that cater to your cravings while protecting your health. Yes, you can still have your favorites.

- **Real-Life Meal Plans**: Includes a 7-Day Meal Plan with recipes to get you started

Don't Just Survive – Thrive!

Say goodbye to the aftermath of dialysis! Discover how a renal diet can improve your life and help you feel your best. Are you ready to elevate your quality of life?

Visit *MagicRecipeCookbook.com* and grab your copy now!

Appendix A: Glossary

Aseptic Technique: Aseptic technique is a set of practices and procedures to prevent contamination from germs and bacteria. Dialysis patients must understand and practice aseptic techniques to minimize the risk of infection during dialysis treatments.

Cannulation: Cannulation is the insertion of a needle into the fistula to establish a connection between the fistula and the dialysis machine. It's necessary for dialysis and must be done carefully, using good aseptic technique, to minimize the risk of infection.

Catheter: A catheter is a tube inserted into a vein or artery for hemodialysis, providing access to the bloodstream for dialysis treatments. For peritoneal dialysis, a catheter is inserted into the belly.

Creatinine[3]: Creatinine is a waste product formed from the digestion of protein in food and the normal breakdown of muscle tissue. It is removed from the blood through your kidneys. Everyone has some creatinine in their blood, but too much can be a sign of a possible kidney problem.

Dialysate: Dialysate is a solution used in dialysis treatments to help remove waste products from the body.

Dialysis Access: Dialysis access is an entry point into your bloodstream used during dialysis treatments. There are different types of access, including fistulas, grafts, and catheters. Fistulas and grafts are surgically created connections between an artery and a vein, allowing blood to be drawn out of and returned to your body during treatment. On the other hand, catheters are tubes inserted directly into a vein in your neck, chest, or groin, providing a temporary access point.

Dialysis Machine: A dialysis machine is a medical device that cleans your blood when your kidneys are unable to do so. It removes toxins, excess fluids, and waste from your blood and then returns the cleaned blood to your body. The machine uses a special dialyzer filter, which works like a sponge to soak up all the bad stuff. It also uses a liquid called dialysate to help with the cleaning process.

Drain Pain: Drain pain refers to the discomfort that can be experienced when your peritoneal catheter removes fluid from the peritoneum during automatic peritoneal dialysis (PD). It may feel like an irritation or a pulling sensation in the abdomen.

Dwell: Dwell is a term used in peritoneal dialysis to describe the time dialysate remains in the patient's abdomen before it is drained.

Electrolytes: Electrolytes help regulate the amount of water in your body and help your cells and organs function properly. Electrolytes are removed from the blood during dialysis. Sodium and potassium are electrolytes.

Fistula: A fistula is a connection between an artery and a vein in your arm or leg, created by a surgeon. It's vital for dialysis because it provides a safe and reliable access point for needles during dialysis treatments.

Hemodialysis: Hemodialysis is a method of cleaning your blood externally through a machine. During the treatment, your blood is taken from your body and passed through a special filter in the dialysis machine, which cleans excess fluids, toxins, and waste that your kidneys can no longer filter out. Once the blood is cleaned, it is returned to your body. Typically, hemodialysis is done three times a week, and each session can take about four hours.

HD: HD stands for hemodialysis, a process that cleans your blood by passing it through a dialyzer, a machine that removes waste products, excess fluids, and electrolytes from your blood.

HHD: HHD stands for home hemodialysis, a type of dialysis performed at home using a machine by the patient alone or with a helper. It can be a more comfortable, convenient, and patient-centered form of dialysis than in-clinic treatments. HHD is much gentler on your body.

Organ Stunning: Organ stunning can occur during hemodialysis, a process in which water is removed too quickly from the blood, resulting in the deprivation of oxygen to organs and tissues.

PD: Stands for peritoneal dialysis

Peritoneal Dialysis: Peritoneal dialysis uses the peritoneum, the lining of the abdomen, as a filter to clean the blood. During treatment, a specific solution is infused into the abdomen through a catheter and left in place for several hours, allowing it to absorb excess fluids, toxins, and waste from the blood. Afterward, the solution is drained out and disposed of. The process can be repeated a few times a day, every day, or on a nightly schedule. The best part is that it can be done at home, giving patients more control over their treatment plan and allowing them to maintain a sense of independence. It's a great alternative to in-center hemodialysis for individuals who prefer a more flexible treatment option.

Residual Function: Residual function is any kidney function a patient has left when they begin dialysis. It's essential to know the level of residual function because it can help determine the frequency of dialysis treatments and the type of dialysis best suited for the patient.

SDHD: SDHD stands for short daily hemodialysis, a type of home hemodialysis done more frequently than regular hemodialysis. It can help improve patients' quality of life by allowing them to spend more time with their families and engage in their usual activities.

Ultrafiltration: Ultrafiltration is a process that is used in hemodialysis treatments to remove excess fluid from the body.

Appendix B
FAQs

Top Questions People Ask When Starting Dialysis

Diet

❦ I'm confused. One site says you can't eat something, while another tells you to limit it.

It's all about how much protein, phosphorus, potassium, sodium, and fluid you consume each day. So if you want to eat a "forbidden" food, then you need to budget for it. Get your daily requirements from your dietitian and view them as a daily food budget. Stick to your daily food budget, and you'll be fine.

❦ How do I lower my potassium?

Many foods contain natural potassium, and most commercially prepared items, such as bread and coffee creamers, contain potassium additives. It is essential to read the ingredients label.

Portion control is the key. You need to know how much potassium you are actually taking in. Look up the nutritional content of your food. Use the _USDA Food Data Central_ (free) or the _Kidney Food Finder_ (small charge) to determine how much potassium you eat or drink.

Weigh your portions and track how much potassium you are consuming daily. Speak to your dietitian to determine your daily limit. My limit was 2,000 mg per day.

☙ (How do I lower my phosphorus?
The answer here is the same as the previous answer. Many foods, especially bakery items, have phosphates added as a preservative.

Read the ingredient label and look for anything that contains "phos." Remember, portion control is essential.

You can look up the phosphorus content of most natural foods in the _USDA Food Database_, (or the _Kidney Food Finder_) but it is generally not available for branded foods. Unfortunately, phosphorus content is not required to be on a food label.

Dialysis

☙ Why do I need dialysis?
Your kidneys are no longer filtering waste and fluid properly. Dialysis does this job for them.

☙ Will I feel tired?
Fatigue is a common but manageable condition that can be alleviated with proper care, rest, and diet.

☙ Will dialysis cure me?
No, dialysis is not a cure; it's a treatment that replaces some of the kidneys' function.

☙ How long will I need it?
Usually, for life, unless you get a kidney transplant or your kidney function improves.

- **What are my options?**
  Hemodialysis: Done at a center or home using a machine.

- *Peritoneal dialysis:* Done at home using your abdominal lining and a machine.

❦ Does it hurt?
The needles may hurt briefly. However, you will usually be given a numbing cream to apply beforehand, and the treatment itself shouldn't be painful.

❦ Can I get a kidney transplant?
Yes, most people can, but be aware, the wait can be several years. Ask your doctor about being added to the transplant list.

❦ How long can I live on dialysis?
Many people live for years. Staying informed and engaged helps improve outcomes.

❦ Can I live a normal life?
Many people still work, travel, and enjoy life on dialysis, with some adjustments.

❦ Can I travel on Dialysis?
Yes!

If you dialyze in-center, work with your clinic. They will arrange for you to be set up with a dialysis clinic at your destination and any stops along the way.

If you dialyze at home, you can bring the machine with you. Your clinic will make arrangements for a backup clinic at your destination(s) to assist you in the event of an emergency.

I once traveled with a PD machine in the car, and it wasn't too bad. The machine was not very heavy. I also traveled once by air with a NxStage Home dialysis machine. That was a little more awkward due to the weight of the machine and the number of supplies to carry.

In both cases, the supplier (Fresenius, NxStage) delivered supplies to my destination.

It was strongly suggested that I carry a 3-day supply with me, which I thought was a good idea.

Please note that airlines are required to accommodate your machine and supplies under the Americans with Disabilities Act (ADA).

It takes some planning, but many people do travel successfully with home equipment.

You will need to coordinate with your clinic, as they will set up a backup clinic at your destination in case you need it. I never needed it.

You'll probably need about three months to contact your supplier, the airline, and your clinic. If you're flying, you'll need a hard case; you should be able to borrow one from your clinic, as they can be expensive. You may want to fly handicapped, especially if you have to change planes and/or terminals.

Bring plenty of $10 bills to tip the porters. You'll probably need them.

Why do I Get Leg Cramps? / Are Leg Cramps Common?
Yes, they are common, but they don't have to be. Leg cramps are usually caused by a deficiency in potassium. Too much potassium can cause cramps, too.

Low potassium levels can be caused by dehydration and/or excessive potassium removal during dialysis. Both often happen at in-center dialysis. When you first start dialysis, a "one size fits all" prescription is usually prescribed. Unless you consult with your kidney doctor, it will likely never change.

Often, one of two things happens: your dry weight is too low, causing excessive fluid removal and leading to dehydration, or the dialysate removes too much potassium. Either, or both, can happen!

In-center dialysis pulls the toxins and fluids off way too fast, causing you to feel lousy.

For all these reasons, I highly recommend home dialysis, which can be either peritoneal dialysis (PD) or Home Hemodialysis. Both are excellent choices, as they are performed more slowly and gently on your body.

Remember, always talk to your kidney doctor and advocate for yourself, because no one else will.

Appendix C
Resources

Along with the insights in this book, I've put together a handy collection of articles, information, and engaging videos that dig deeper into dialysis and the renal diet. To access all these valuable links in one convenient place, simply visit:

https://kidneydietcentral.com/get-resources/.

Jump in and give yourself the knowledge and tools you need to not only survive but *THRIVE!*

KidneyDietCentral.com

Learn how to follow a renal diet WITHOUT giving up your favorite food. Discover the different types of dialysis and determine which one is right for you. *https://KidneyDietCentral.com*

Facebook

On dialysis? Wondering what to do or what to eat? You have found the right place. We talk about the kidney diet, what it is, and how it relates to dialysis. We also discuss the different types of dialysis. *https://www.facebook.com/KidneyDietCentral/*

Appendix D: Endnotes

[1] Harvard Medical School (2017, January 23). Potassium lowers blood pressure. Harvard Health Publishing. Retrieved February 13, 2025, from *https://www.health.harvard.edu/heart-health/potassium-lowers-blood-pressure#:~:text=Normal%20body%20levels%20of%20potassium,and%20higher%20risk%20of%20stroke*

[2] Timothy Jee Kam Koh Nocturnal hemodialysis: improved quality of life and patient outcomes. National
Library of Medicine National Center for Biotechnology Information Pubmed Central
Published online 2019 Apr 3. doi: 10.2147/IJNRD.S165919 Available at *https://www.ncbi.nlm.nih.gov/pmc/articles/PMC6452820/*

[3] National Kidney Foundation (2023, June 1). Creatinine. Retrieved February 13, 2025, from *https://www.kidney.org/kidney-topics/creatinine#:~:text=More%20resources,About%20Creatinine,of%20a%20possible%20kidney%20problem*

www.ingramcontent.com/pod-product-compliance
Lightning Source LLC
Chambersburg PA
CBHW070257290326
41930CB00041B/2625